I0407811

Also by Dr. Stenbeck

Available from the usual on-line source

Books

Healing Yourself -- The Holistic Approach
   [An introduction to Holistic Self-healing.]

Heal Yourself Right Now!
   [The Seven Priority Organ Levels for
   effective Nutritional/Holistic Treatment of
   all organs.]

The 22 Unique Body Types
   (for Health and Weight Loss)
Q & A to Identify Your Body Type
   [Individual Type booklets are also available

Booklets
(Step-by-step instructions on healing yourself)

   #1 *Start Healing with Positive Thinking*
   #2 *Mastering Positive Feelings for Health!*
   #3 *Spiritual Balance and Your Healing*

The Myogenic Body Type

The President Bill Clinton, Julia Roberts Celebrity Body Type

For Kaye,
there at the beginning with Doc Severn,
and for Liberty,
continuing the holistic healing journey...

Disclaimer

The information in this book is for educational purposes only and is not a substitute for medication, diets, or other medical care. The diets do not treat diseases or medical conditions, and are an adjunct to your orthodox health care.

The author and publisher accept no responsibility for any misuse of the information within. If you have any physical problem, food allergy, emotional disorder, or disease, common sense dictates that you consult with a physician before changing your diet, taking nutritional supplements, or following the advice given here.

———

About the Author

Educated in New Zealand and in the U.S.A., Dr. Stenbeck attained B.Sc. (NZ), M.S., and D.C. degrees. His holistic healing methods have been profiled in magazines (Esquire, McLean's, Playgirl, the Atlanta Constitution), and on TV in the USA and in Canada. He was the main contributor to the Warner Book, _The Eye/Body Connection_ by Jessica Maxwell that focused on the holistic healing relationships between the iris structure and organ genetics.

In the 1970-80's he was elected Fellow, Royal Society of Health, London; Fellow, American Association of Chemists; Member, American Association of Clinical Chemists; and Affiliate, Royal Society of Medicine, London. He studied naturopathy and Body Types with Dr. Bernard Jensen and Dr. Clifford Severn, and has practiced in medical partnerships where patients received the joint benefits of medical and holistic healing.

He is a member of Self-Realization Fellowship. To receive advice on any health issue from a holistic viewpoint, or to receive help with your body type, see his web site: *DrStenbeck.net*

———

Contents

* * *

The Myogenic Body Type and Food Guide   *1*

* * *

The 22 Body Types:
Celebrity Examples

This Booklet contains the **Myogenic** type. See
<u>The 22 Unique Body Types</u> for all type
descriptions.]

Thin Types

Atrophic   *Woody Allen / Audrey Hepburn*
              Stan Laurel / Calista Flockheart

Exesthesic   *Cher / Sarah Jessica Parker*
              (Female type only)

Marasmic   *President Obama / Princess Diana*
              James Stewart / Kate Blanchard

Neurogenic   *J.K. Simmons / Joan Rivers*
              Jon Cryer / Marin Hinle

Pathoferic   *(No celebrity males)*
              Blythe Danner / Gwyneth Paltrow

Sillevitic   *David Bowie / Shirley MacLaine*
              Rod Stewart / Carol Channing

Muscle Types

Calciferic	*Michael Jordan / Angelica Huston* *Abraham Lincoln / Grace Jones*
Carbogenic	*George Clooney / Lady Gaga* *Pres. G. Bush, Jr. / Meg Ryan*
Desmogenic	*Marlon Brando / Loni Anderson* *Daniel Craig / Tina Turner*
Eldic	*Ross Perot / Hillary Clinton* *Peter Falk / Sigourney Weaver*
Myogenic	*Pres. Bill Clinton / Sharon Stone* *Pres. John Kennedy / Julia Roberts*
Nervimotive	*Frank Sinatra / Elizabeth Taylor* *Mark Wahlberg / Natalie Wood*
Nitropheric	*Ben Affleck / Ava Gardner* *Kirk Douglas / Kate Winslet*
Pallinomic	*Pres. Donald Trump /* *Attorney General Janet Reno* *Bill O'Reilly (Fox) / Jane Russell*

Fat Types

Barotic Robin Williams / "Mrs.Doubtfire"
          Elton John / William Conrad

Carboferic Bill Murray / Roseanne
             Billy Gardell / Melissa McCarthy

Hydripheric John Goodman / Shelly Winters
              Wayne Knight / Jennifer Holliday

Isogenic Einstein / Oprah Winfrey
           Phillip S .Hoffman / Queen Victoria

Lipopheric Rush Limbaugh / Rosie O'Donnell
             Chris Christie / Camryn Manheim

Oxypheric Winston Churchill / Orsen Welles
            Ella Fitzgerald / Gerry Spence

Pargenic Burt Reynolds / Katey Segal
           Ron Perlman / Kirstey Alley

Succinct Quote on Human Types

From Victor Rocine, who first described discrete body types around 1900.

"A type is an order of people that differentiates and distinguishes itself by a general and similar form, brain-formation, chemistry, structure, build, immunity, tendencies, predisposition, resemblance, skin-pigment, and type characteristics based on observation and analogy.

"Or, in other words, people of a given type are similar physically and like-minded as if they were brothers and sisters—that is what type means.

"Everything in nature is made according to plan. Man only discovers that plan and gives it a name. The zoologist has not made the animals—he has only described the plan adopted by the wonderful Creator, and named the classes, sub-classes, etc.

"How important type research will be to humanity, time alone will make known."

———

Prologue

The esteemed scientist J. J. Berzelius, discoverer of several chemical elements, inspired Victor Rocine to research body types and to investigate the correlation between types and their diseases. Around 1890-1910, Rocine privately published his original findings on the mineral basis of different body types, and this present book exists because of his brilliant insights.

For many years, I studied with Dr. Clifford Severn who had been a personal student of Victor Rocine on body types, naturopathy, herbology, iris analysis, diet, and nutritional healing methods. He had a successful career as a lecturer and healer, and was one of those rare athletes with complete muscle control over his body. I saw him under a spotlight at 85 years of age, contracting and rippling every individual muscle in his perfectly developed body. Field-Marshal Jan Smuts, the WWII South African Prime Minister, devoted a full chapter of his autobiography to how Severn's healing methods had saved his life. In the 1950's, *Life* magazine did a four-page spread on Severn and his family. Fame he had.

Another Rocine student I studied with, Dr. Bernard Jensen wrote of Rocine's body type research and nutritional methods in his privately published book *The Chemistry of Man*.

This book is deeply rooted in Rocine's original work, and with that of Herbert Shelton, M.D., Ph.D. (at Harvard University in the 1930's). I integrated their research with newer dietary and nervous system data along with celebrity examples of each type, hopefully, making this material easier to digest and more entertaining for the reader.

Gayelord Hauser, another Rocine student I knew, was a celebrated health book author. He wrote a popular book on Rocine's types in the 1940's, *Types and Temperaments;* reputedly, he also introduced yogurt to the western world.

This book exists because of Rocine's creative brilliance and original discoveries in natural healing.

▶ *Rocine: "The soul creates the body type."*

Rocine taught that the soul chooses a body type and brain to live in, thus presenting different experiences and life lessons to master. Why were *you* born the way you are?

That is something to think about, especially if it is true! What would your soul purpose be to live in a particular body type. I provide some thoughts on this issue in each type description and try to assess from my experience with your type the particular lessons of life presented therein.

Rocine was as brilliant in his way as an Abraham Lincoln, Michael Jordan, Michael Phelps, Tony Robbins, or a Daniel Day Lewis—all *calciferic* types—rare, leaders, innovative, brilliant, and highly intelligent in their different fields of endeavor.

Celebrity examples exist for most types, not a duplicate of you, but someone who has your essence in their body-mind individuality. Knowing your type allows you to become a better you!

The celebrity examples provide further help in identifying your body type.

▶ *Rocine's classic findings are the backbone of this book. Integrated with Sheldon's research and with other dietary and food issues including mental, emotional, and spiritual attributes,*

Many people take nutritional supplements and try different diets without a doctor's advice. If this is your choice, use common sense, listen to body responses, and discontinue any allergic reactions to foods or nutritional substances.

———

The Myogenic Body Type

Representing one of the 22 Body Types first described by Victor Rocine around 1900

* * *

"You may also have a physical or psychological feature not representative of your type such as height, weight, appearance, talent, weakness, strength, etc., due to biochemical errors, environmental influences, racial or cultural differences, and congenital or genetic issues. Nevertheless, the type identification of the average person is usually clear."

— *Victor Rocine*

Myogenic Type Celebrity Examples

*If you think this is your type, be sure to look at **on-line photographs** of these examples. Look for general similarities to yourself. Note that sub-types cause the differences in appearance between members of the same type.*

————

GOVERNMENT

President Bill Clinton
President Franklin Roosevelt
President Kennedy
Vice President Nelson Rockefeller
Senator Ted Kennedy
Senator Robert Kennedy
Senator John Lindsay

NOTABLES

Jackie Kennedy   Carolyn Kennedy
John F. Kennedy, Jr.   Princess Grace

ACTORS

Clark Gable   Omar Sharif
Robert Redford   Paul Newman
Jeffrey Hunter   Brandon Fraser

Henry Cavill, Christopher Reeve (both as "Superman")

And the beautiful ladies…

Julia Roberts	Jane Fonda
Diana Riggs	Katherine Ross
Charlize Theron	Cameron Diaz
Glenda Jackson	Michelle Pfeiffer
Daryl Hannah	Faye Dunaway
Christie Brinkley	Lauren Hutton
Jacqueline Bisset	Ann Bancroft
Muriel Hemingway	Lindsay Wagner
Catherine Deneuve	Eva Marie Saint
Ali McGraw	Farrah Fawcett
Brook Shields	Susan Anton
Lauren Bacall	Charmian Carr
Blair Brown	Tanya Roberts

TV

Ted Koppel	Bill Kurtis (A&E)
Sean Hannity	Megan Kelly

VOICE

Jack Jones	Pat Boone
Steve Lawrence	
Olivia Newton-John	Debby Boone

SPORTS

Jerry West	Gail Goodrich
Pat Haden	Arnold Palmer
John Elway	Steve Garvey

Jack Nicholas (many pro golfers)

OLYMPICS

Bart Connor (U.S.A. Gold medalist)
Bruce Jenner (U.S.A. Gold medalist)
Peter Snell (N.Z. Gold medalist)
John Walker (N.Z. Gold medalist)

ARTS

Margot Fontaine (ballet)
(Many top fashion models are this type.)

OTHER (from Rocine)

Jack London	Shakespeare

[I personally knew one of the above celebrities, many other examples in everyday life and in my family, which contributed to my understanding of the type.]

Read the types, and if still confused you may choose to use the personal request for type identification from the web site: *DrStenbeck.net*

―――――

Myogenic Type Questionnaire

Other than for the physical descriptions, these questions describe the generic type, and not specifically you! If any question ever applied to you, then choose the True answer!

For Question 1 only:

A = True	B = Maybe	C = Untrue
15 points	7 points	1 point

1. Physically identify with a celebrity   _____

Then...

A = True	B = Maybe	C = Untrue
5 points	3 points	1 point

---

2. Height is close to:
   Males: 5'6-6'4   Females: 5'4-6'1   _____
3. Usual weight is close to:
   Males: 160-250   Females: 110-175   _____
4. Females shapely; males muscular   _____
5. Medium-sized (some heavier)   _____
6. Females emotional and reactive; males
   calm, poised, controlled   _____
7. Naturally friendly, happy, outgoing   _____
8. Hair full, thick, fine, wavy, all colors   _____
9. Males handsome; females, attractive or
   beautiful   _____

10. Male chest is full, some quite hairy;
    female bust small, some medium-sized ____
11. Intelligent, good intellect, debating ability;
    academically accomplished, often brilliant ____
12. Low impulse control creates life problems ____
13. Some desire alcohol, nicotine, drugs; some
    females vulnerable to eating disorders ____
14. Excellent judges of character (and
    make fine judges) ____
15. Highly developed social skills,
    communicators, congenial ____
16. Natural managers, organizers, planners ____
17. Idealistic, sympathetic, always help others ____
18. Are very outgoing and popular ____
19. Happy, optimistic ____
20. Pleasant, friendly, and influential ____
21. May rebel against the establishment ____
22. Satirical sense of humor ____
23. Enjoy speaking, teaching, performing,
    singing, influencing people; a strong voice ____
24. Strong sexual drive; some are impulsive ____
25. Observe, listen, have common sense ____
26. Management, sports, communing abilities ____
27. Imaginative; ambitious, enterprising ____
28. Talents in business, sales, public relations,
    diplomacy, banking, negotiations, writing,
    acting, athletics, executives, lecturing,
    teaching, speech, medicine ____
29. Dislike 'hard' sales; cannot stretch truth ____
30. Arms and legs lean, strong, proportional
    in females; males are muscular ____
31. Desire beef (limit it after age 40 for health) ____
32. Very able in finance, sports, healing work ____
33. Tolerant of others opinions, poised ____

34. Empathetic and sympathetic to others _____
35. Able to eloquently express self; stubbornly defend point of view _____
36. Feelings easily hurt in love relationships _____
37. Have deep respect and love of family _____
38. Deep sense of truth, honesty, ethics _____
39. Are cool in emergencies _____
40. Have a genuine love of people _____
41. Magnetic, popular, friendly, optimistic _____
42. Love ecology and/or animals (like *eldics*) _____
43. Animated, magnetic, engaging gestures _____
44. Males gain fat easily (with a fat sub-type); eating disorders in some females _____
45. Greet people like friends; greetings real and honest; handshake strong, sincere _____
46. Head proportional, attractive, balanced; top-head usually high and rounded _____
47. Blue or brown eyes; vision weak _____
48. Normal-sized ears (except with *eldic* sub-type); good hearing _____
49. If in a position of power, commitments are honored _____
50. Dispense equal justice; fair, honest _____
51. Have balanced and attractive lips _____
52. May have excessive tolerance of others' behaviors _____
53. Muscles prominent; strong, lean _____
54. Muscular, broad, strong back and shoulders _____
55. Strong flexible joints; some double-jointed _____
56. Many liberal, democratic (many feminists) _____
57. May have moral weakness _____

58. Face attractive, curved cheekbones, nice features; vertical on profile view; strong lower jaw (especially males) _____
59. Highly social; communicate with anyone; strong sales ability based on honesty _____
60. Strong belief in God; have spiritual or metaphysical beliefs _____
61. Unselfish; ambitious to help mankind _____
62. May have excessive sympathy for others _____
63. Are brave, fearless and courageous after assessing risks _____

Scoring

For question #1:
A response: give 15 points   = _____
B response: give 7 points   = _____
C response: give 1 points   = _____

For questions #2—63:
A response: give 5 points   = _____
B response: give 3 points   = _____
C response: give 1 point   = _____

Total of the above points   = _____

Interpretation
160—295: PROBABLY Myogenic
80—159: POSSIBLY Myogenic
<80: NOT Myogenic

The Myogenic Type

Rocine: "Myogenic means 'muscle producing'. Compared to other types, myogenics are more balanced in physique, limb, and brain." You utilize more food potassium than most types, which helps calcium and mineral absorption, and contributes to balanced muscle and brain development.

———

Myogenics have a natural musculature, obvious in males like Robert Redford, Christopher Reeve, and Clark Gable, but less obvious in females (who nevertheless are strong). The females are lean, shapely, pretty, or beautiful, and small-busted (Megan Kelly, Grace Kelly). The tall fashion models are invariably your type, whereas the *myogenics* seen in everyday life are mostly medium-sized. You are calm under pressure, poised and non-excitable; some females are more emotionally reactive, but reliable in emergencies.

▶ *The males may easily hold fat (if either parent is a fat type). Parents of a myogenic must watch teen years for eating and behavioral disorders, smoking, drugs, and alcohol abuse, which commonly happens!*

———

Physical Similarity to Other Types

The *nitropheric* type (Harrison Ford, Jessica Lange) is similarly built, but more withdrawn and private.

The younger male *oxypheric* type (Winston Churchill, Ella Fitzgerald) is fleshier with a larger head.

The female *eldic* (Nancy Reagan) and *desmogenic* (Loni Anderson) types may appear similar except for freckles, and often being natural redheads.

The male *desmogenic* (Val Kilmer, Daniel Craig) may look similar, but has a square jaw, and is more intense and forceful.

———

Average Height and Weight

Males:	5'6-6'4	160-250
Females:	5'4-6'1	110-175

You already know something about this type from their public persona and appearance, whether from seeing them yourself or from the celebrity examples. Blend such insights with the type descriptions and types of your family and friends to discern their presence in your midst!

———

Myogenic Type Description

The type description represents how you appear in everyday society. You may have a sub-type that alters parts of this description.

Think of the celebrity examples as you read the descriptions. You show markedly short and tall varieties in both sexes; for example, the tall Christopher Reeve, compared to the shorter Ted Koppel (ABC) and Bob Costas (NBC). If male, you are well muscled with an attractive or handsome face and body; the body is often hairy, but not excessively so like the *carbogenic, nervimotive, and pargenic* types. The female is shapely, attractive or beautiful, and never plain. Quite a few are tomboys when younger. Every *myogenic* female I have known has been handsome, pretty, or beautiful. There are more "drop-dead" beautiful females of this type compared to all other types! Your minds are better than average, many being superior.

Head — Your head is proportional, attractive, and balanced in size; the forehead is usually high (like the *oxypheric*); the backhead is often high and rounded as in Clark Gable and Christopher Reeve.

Hair — The hair is full, fine, wavy, and dry, in all colors; if blonde, you are bright and intelligent!

Eyes — Blue or brown colors are usual; some visual weakness may be present; the eyebrows are curved and bushy in many males (Brendan Fraser).

Ears — Your hearing sense is well developed. Normal-sized ears are common except when an *eldic* sub-type is present as in Clark Gable who had large floppy ears (before the studios pinned them back). Shorter muscular and handsome males with large ears like Ross Perot and Dustin Hoffman are invariably *eldic*.

Nose — You have a balanced nose.

Face — The face is usually straight up and down on profile; the lower jaw is long and strong.

► *Your face is attractive and balanced, with gentle curving cheek-bones, and a square-rectangular look from the front.*

Mouth and Lips — Your lips are balanced and attractive, while your voice is pleasant, friendly, influential, and strong. You are good talkers and can communicate with anyone.

Teeth — The teeth are white, normal-sized, and usually strong, although a few have weak calcium metabolism.

Skin — As teenagers, your intake of cigarettes, pot, sugar, fast foods and drugs may initiate acne, giving way to attractive skin as adults (when healthy).

Neck — Your neck is muscular and normal-sized.

Muscles — The muscles are prominent, but not as strong as the *lipopheric, carbogenic, desmogenic, and pallinomic* types whose muscle development is greater than their bone formation. Moderate exercise is essential to your health. Your body, built on efficiency rather than brute strength, is never seen in weight-lifting or body building competitions since you crave movement over static sports. Your type, found in professional sports, win many Olympic Gold medals.

Chest — If male, your chest is large with light to medium hair growth. The female bust is invariably small, some of moderate size.

▶ *Breast augmentation may make typing confusing (many Playboy centerfolds). A beautiful, lean, small busted, shapely woman is usually your type.*

Back and Shoulders — The back and shoulders are muscular, broad and strong in males, and more balanced in females.

Abdomen and Hips — The abdomen and hips are medium-sized with an average waistline; the males often become heavier around the mid-section.

Arms and Legs — Your extremities are proportional. The hands are often muscular with medium-sized fingernails. Shorter females may have larger calves and thighs. Your gestures (like the *oxypheric*) are animated, magnetic and engaging; when others first meet you they feel like your long lost friend; your handshake and greetings are strong, honest, sincere, and friendly.

Joints — Strong and flexible joints characterize your type with many USA Olympic gymnasts. (Note that European countries tend to have male *desmogenics* as their star gymnasts while Asian countries have more *nervimotives*.)

———

Myogenic Personality Traits

If you are this Muscle type many, but not all, of the following characteristics are present. You may have overcome or moderated the negatives, but also recognize that you may have once had them.

You may have any of the following traits:

- Have utopian views
- Unselfish in helping others
- May be feminists (like *eldics*)
- Love outdoor life and nature
- Friendly, satiric sense of humor
- Assertive, but may become aggressive
- A strong sales ability based on honesty
- High inquisitiveness, always seeking data
- Usually positive, hopeful about the future
- Love travel and pleasure; genuinely desire to help people
- Love sporting activities, nature, camping, outdoors, etc.
- If in a position of power, equal justice is dispensed to all
- You are powerful in honest social interaction with anyone
- You are able to see all sides of an issue and make fair judgments; are attracted to criminal law

- Usually don't care about money or status, but may become rich through your talents; are ambitious
- You have an enviable ability to talk to anyone, anywhere, in an open, honest, and engaging manner
- Others may disagree with your choices, but you always try to fulfill your promises; you live your truth
- Are carefully brave by assessing risks and then taking action (unlike the *desmogenic* who jumps right in)
- Attitude is positive and friendly unless emotionally scarred in childhood in which case you appear neutral
- High social skills: you are able to commune sincerely with anyone from a pauper to a king, as evident in Presidents' Kennedy, Clinton
- Have strong beliefs in God or meta-physics; many are attracted to the ministry; have a strong relationship with God; many active in church activities
- Are in control of your emotions; even if upset, you may not show it; sooner or later, the anxious *myogenic* female explodes; the male is more controlled
- Your brain is powerful with many of you gaining high academic honors,

doctorates, etc. (President Bill Clinton won an esteemed Rhodes Scholarship)

- Have a balanced mind without any excessively strong or weak brain centers; are born leaders, organizers, managers, strategic officers in time of war; although capable, hand to hand combat is not your choice; you have a high ability to convince and influence other people

▶ *Rocine: "You are the 'salt of the earth'…but you love to eat, drink, and be merry. You may be out-of-control, over-do it, and ruin your career through errors of commission."*

Potential Challenges

You may have evolved from, or not experienced these general challenges, so do not dwell on them.

▶ *Rocine: "Some myogenics are weak in honesty, ethics, and duty, resulting in vanity and self-indulgence. You have mental weaknesses and are not as moral as some types. Myogenic faults are no worse than any other type, and are perhaps less than most."*

- May spend more than is available

- May desire nicotine, alcohol, or drugs in teen years
- Some have morality issues (Kennedy family, Bill Clinton, etc.); have an excellent ability to stretch the truth
- Have excessive sympathy and empathy with others' problems (inappropriate compassion and tolerance)
- Low self-esteem and other self-negative feelings are common; some females may enter co-dependent relationships

---

Myogenic Stress Management

You have strong mental stress prevention giving you a good ability not to internalize this stress into your stomach, adrenals, and immune system. Emotional stress prevention is variable, and any of the above challenges may need reprogramming help. *(If needing help managing these stresses, see my prior books.)*

Love

A strong and urgent sexual drive is usual (some examples have a carnal nature). You are attracted to lean or medium-sized types and may fall in love and marry suddenly with miserable results from such unions! You tend to mate with the *nitropheric, carbogenic, pathoferic, and eldic* types.

———

Talents and Vocations

Abilities - *Management, executives, finance, sports, medicine, teaching, commerce, negotiations, journalism, diplomacy, teaching, psychology, science, public relations, stock-markets, show business*

You are ambitious, enterprising, successful, excellent students, and like the *calciferic* type you learn by observation and listening. Speech, expression, talking, and negotiation are your greatest talents. You have many talents, but wasted teen years and rebelliousness may cause you to drop out of high school. You are often tempted into alcohol, drug, or sexual experimentation. Politics is a natural for you. In observing President Clinton and the Kennedy family one sees how cleverly you blend the game of politics and mass communication with an honest view of the truth.

▶ *I have known or observed you as bankers, physicians, actors, entrepreneurs, singers, models, dancers, holistic healers, seminar leaders, high school dropouts, and as executives.*

Inabilities - *Law, "hard" sales*

You are not usually attracted to occupations requiring confrontation, but if required you can confront with the best of them! If a lawyer, you may enter government service. The type information cannot predict what or who you will become, but you are capable of bringing a creative excellence or brilliance to whatever you do in life.

———

Health Problems

Myogenics have good resistance to disease, your genetics being stronger than most types. If sick, you commonly experience health problems or diseases in any of the following areas:

Eyes — The eyes are weak and easily strained.

Lungs — The lungs are weak and vulnerable.

Liver — Alcohol or drug intake commonly damages the liver.

Skin — There is a vulnerability to acne and minor skin problems.

Joints — Aches and pains are common in females (usually allergies).

Nerves — The nerves, easily exhausted, make you irritable and impatient; the females are prone to emotional outbursts.

Heart and Circulatory System — Males may over-indulge in exercise, with excessive red meat intake causing heart enlargement; you need moderate exercise and a low beef intake.

Myogenic Acid/Alkaline Factor

[See the Appendix for details on this subject, along with the common symptoms found with people of different nervous system dominance.]

For your health and healing, the genetics of your autonomic nervous system predispose you to needing a specific ratio of food acidity to alkalinity. You are born with an ***intermediate*** constitution, which means you need a balance between acid and alkaline-ash foods in your diet. (Ash refers to the minerals left in your body after metabolizing foods. Your autonomic nervous system genetics are intermediate between the *parasympathetic* and *sympathetic* nervous systems, making this acid/alkaline question less important for you compared to the predominantly acid and alkaline types.

50% Fruits, salads, vegetables
50% Proteins, carbohydrates

▶ *Approximate your food ratios. On any particular day, it does not matter if one meal is mostly alkaline and another mostly acid—just try to balance it out for the day! If you make a mistake, try again tomorrow. It is a subjective call that you make, as what you do over weeks and months makes the difference to your health.*

The Myogenic Spiritual Factor

Skip this paragraph if uninterested in a philosophical perspective on your body type!

▶ *Rocine: "The soul chooses the body type."*

If as souls, we choose the brain and body type to spend a lifetime in, it could be to learn certain spiritual lessons related to perfecting ourselves, and our humanity, in God's eyes. What lessons does the type bring you? Only you can really decide what those lessons are. You know your weaknesses, faults, and behaviors towards others. You know things about yourself that Victor Rocine could never get from his research subjects when he first wrote about types. So search your mind for the answers.

Each discrete type has challenges of life lessons, spiritual goals, etc., and some of yours may be:

Over-reliance on Personal Power — You readily attract people into your life—both good and bad. Not being so trusting is an important lesson.

Low Will-power — You may lack the will to accomplish goals, which feeds your negative impulse control. Affirmations and therapy helps.

Impulse Control — Giving in to your impulses may cause you to hurt yourself or others. Learning how to control them is important for your happiness.

Addiction — In teen years, you are vulnerable to alcohol, drugs, sex, and smoking: strong parental influence and psychological counseling keeps you on track.

———

A Myogenic Story…

Danny, age 24, 5'6, fair-haired, blue-eyes and handsome, was congenial and sociable. He complained of fatigue, headaches, moods, nervousness, indigestion, and increased weight.

Examination revealed good health with diet being the major problem. He ate excessive carbon foods: sugars, fats, starches, dried fruits, and cereals and breads; he also ate excessive salty junk foods: catsup, preserved meats, canned meats, peanut butter, barbecue sauce, canned and frozen vegetables.

His diet was deficient in the trace minerals (especially iodine), and one or two daily servings of the following foods were keys to his healing: artichokes, kelp, nuts, clams, parsley, whole grains, cod liver oil, spinach (fresh), raisins, turnip greens, and rhubarb.

Danny made these dietary changes, and took the herbs indicated for his type. His symptoms steadily resolved.

Note -

The following recommendations are for the generic type. Additionally, you may need from a holistic healer or nutritionist something more specific for your individuality.

———

Myogenic Type Mineral Foods

Apply this mineral data to the diet following these Muscle type descriptions.

Excessive Foods:

- *Carbon (simple carbohydrates)*
- *Iron*
- *Sodium (salt, salted junk foods)*
- *Nitrogen (red meats)*

Deficient Foods:

- *Potassium*
- *Calcium*
- *Trace Minerals*
- *Sodium (unsalted, non-junk)*
- *Nitrogen (vegetarian sources)*

These deficient minerals are common deficiencies in your type, predisposing you to ill-health; eat these foods daily. (If not ill, eat them 3-4 times weekly.) The lists are in descending order of concentration; choose food servings in the upper half of each list first!
One serving is ½ cup (minimum).

Myogenic Excessive Foods -

Carbon is often excessive so minimize its intake. It is excessive in all people who become fat or obese, and is in every cell of your body as the basis of life. You are not a Fat type, but can pack it on if not careful! Avoid dairy foods, simple carbohydrates, corn syrup, and white sugar foods.

Iron tends to be excessive in your tissues. Do not take mineral tablets that contain iron (unless blood tests prove you have anemia)!

Sodium from salted junk foods is excessive in your tissues. To preserve your health and weight control you should avoid junk foods and fulfill your sodium needs from the food list (without using the salt-shaker).

Nitrogen from red meat is excessive in your diet (if eaten more than twice monthly), and is a major cause of your acidity and illnesses.

———

Deficient Foods –

In illness or disease, it is important to correct these deficiencies.

Potassium is deficient in your type. It is concentrated in and vital to the health of your muscles, heart, brain and all cells. If ill or diseased, potassium foods (and supplements) may be a significant healing factor.

Calcium is deficient and you thrive on dairy foods. It is highly concentrated in bones, joints, muscles, nerves, heart, teeth, and gums; if you have an illness or disease in any of these tissues calcium foods and supplements may be a significant healing factor.

Trace Minerals easily become deficient in your type due to emotional stress or poor digestion and absorption.

Sodium in food form is deficient (see above note).

Nitrogen from vegetable sources is deficient. Some of you choose strict vegetarianism, and a daily powdered protein drink is then essential for your protein balance.

———

Minimize
Excessive Foods

Carbon, Iron: *1-2 servings/week only*

Simple sugars, fats, starches, sweet fruits, dried fruits, legumes, shell-fish, molasses, blackberries, liver, organ meats, deep-green leafy vegetables, asparagus, spinach, prunes (and avoid iron skillets).

Sodium (salted, junk): *0-1 servings/week*

Salt, all fast foods, packaged foods, canned and frozen foods, soy sauce, all preserved meats (cured, smoked, canned and luncheon meats), sauces (barbecue, catsup, etc.), dill pickles, sauerkraut, bouillon cubes, peanut butter, potato chips, etc., salted nuts, crackers, canned or packaged soups, processed cheeses, commercial salad dressings, meat tenderizers.
Note: If you should eat anything on this list, keep it down to 0-1 times weekly!

Nitrogen (beef):

Beef, red meats: 0-2 days <u>monthly</u>

Eat
Deficient Foods

Potassium, Calcium: *1-2 servings/day*

Dulse, kelp, brewer's yeast, whole rice, sunflower seeds, almonds, Swiss and cheddar cheese, turnip greens, corn tortillas, dandelion greens, banana, baked potato with skin, raisins, parsley, un-hulled sesame seeds, Brazil nuts, ripe olives, alfalfa, tofu, watercress, buttermilk, yogurt, tomatoes, berries.

Trace Minerals: *1-2 servings/day*

Parsley, nuts, whole grains (limited), kelp, artichokes, Brazil nuts, brewer's yeast, broccoli, brown rice, cod liver oil, raisins, turnip greens, chicken, garlic, onions, vegetables, rhubarb, green soup, salmon (limited), mushrooms, Irish moss.

Sodium (unsalted, non-junk):
   1-2 servings/day

Kelp, olives, cheddar cheese, cottage cheese, Swiss chard, beets and tops, buttermilk, celery, poultry (3 times/week), sesame seeds, watercress, turnips, carrots, yogurt, parsley.
Note: Use the salt-shaker sparingly!

Eat…

Nitrogen (vegetable):

Peas, beans, black-eyed peas, seeds, nuts, pasta, spirulina —as desired

Eggs, poultry, fish —3-4 days weekly

Note: *Eat any healthy foods you desire, but be sure to include the type foods in your daily choices.*

Myogenic Nutritional Supplements

- **Multi-Vitamins** —
  [Take all supplements with food]
  2 capsules/day
- **Potassium** —
  99 mg/day
- **Calcium** —
  600 mg/twice daily
- **Manganese** —
  50 mg/day
- **Pantothenic Acid** —
  500 mg/twice daily
- **Herbs** —
  Brain detox – Vervain or Gotu Kola
  Organ detox – Fo-ti or Milk Thistle
  (Take one capsule, twice daily for one
  month; then one, three times weekly.)

- **Lecithin** —
  1,300 mg/three times weekly

- **Evening Primrose or Flaxseed Oil**
  1 soft-gel/day with food.
  Note: Be sure to take these supplements if
  you have ill-health.

Important Myogenic Health Concerns

You need meats (limited beef), poultry, fish, potassium foods, green salads, and vegetables in your diet; your genetics require the *Muscle Type* Food Guide for health and any flesh cravings are normal and healthy for you. After about age 50, you need less beef and four or more vegetarian days each week.

▶ *Rocine: "You should eat vegetable protein sources daily, and minimize dairy products and beef."*

Although many *myogenic* women choose semi-vegetarianism, the male's love of beef often precludes this beneficial happening. Meat eating, especially beef, is a major health problem in adult males.

Dairy allergy is common and calcium should be obtained from green leafy vegetables, citrus fruits and juices. Other possible allergies are to wheat, grains, sugar, alcohol, and high-fructose corn syrups.

———

<u>*Myogenic Food Guide*</u>

Aim for –
50% Proteins, complex carbohydrates
50% Fruits, salads, vegetables
and
50% Raw food diet
50% Cooked foods

Lose the salt-shaker
Avoid dairy products
Take the recommended supplements.

Myogenic Weight Loss

Losing weight depends upon you following the type instructions, summarized in this section. Usually you have little trouble losing extra weight by reducing calorie intake and by exercising. However, if desiring to lose weight:

- *Stop* eating junk sodium foods (see list)
- *Protein* drink daily, have about 25-30 grams
- *Eat* your body type deficient mineral foods daily
- *Follow* your *Myogenic Guide (as above)*

- *Exercise*: your body type requires moderate daily exercise
- *Simple sugars*: stop all white table sugar and high-fructose corn syrup and drinks containing these sugars
- *Hypoglycemia:* this hormonal imbalance stops fat loss, and usually initiates more fat production, so if you have this problem it is vital to deal with it: take *pantothenic acid,* 500 mg/twice daily with food (see my earlier books to resolve this problem)
- *Calories:* As with any dietary approach, calories in, must be *less than* calories out! Most markets sell a calorie booklet; make notes of your daily intake, and in most instances keep it under about 1500 calories/day

———

A Food Guide follows for semi-carnivores, the myogenic type having such genes, but a semi-vegetarian diet is more appropriate for health, and often is intuitively desired.

———

Muscle Types
General Food Guide

(Carnivores)

Important Note

———

The Food Guide addresses the <u>Acid-Alkaline</u> aspect of your food intake, along with the <u>Type Mineral</u> factor presented throughout this book. It does <u>not</u> necessarily address calories or other dietary factors that may be pertinent to your personal health needs whether medical or appropriate for some other dietary need. So use your common sense and just include the factors described here with whatever healthy dietary choices you usually make.

For other nutrient information, consult with nutritional books or with holistic nutritional doctors. I particularly recommend the advice of Andrew Weil, M.D.

———

Muscle Types
General Food Guide

(Not for the Nitropheric Type)

*This chapter presents a **general** Food Guide: superimpose on it the nutritional information from your type chapter. As a Muscle body type, your genetics require flesh foods. (Note that a Thin sub-type would move you towards being vegetarian.)*

———

Meat/Flesh Intake

Most muscle types should limit red meat to once or less weekly, while eggs, lamb, fish, or poultry are excellent in moderation. If ill or diseased, be sure to eat daily, one or two servings from each *deficient minerals* list. If not ill, eat them at least three times weekly for health maintenance. If this diet is similar to your present diet, but healing is sluggish, then:

- Decrease your carbohydrate and protein intake by about one-third
- Increase your fruit, salad, and vegetable intake by about one-third
- Consult with a holistic doctor, preferably one versed in nutritional and emotional evaluation

———

Over-Acid or Over-Alkaline?

Just as a log of wood burned in your fireplace leaves a mineral-ash, food ash refers to the minerals remaining after metabolizing foods in your tissues:

- Fruits, vegetables **alkalinize** tissues
- Proteins, carbohydrates **acidify** tissues

Usually You Are Over-Acid Due To:

- Excessive intake: dairy foods
- Excessive intake: proteins, carbohydrates
- Deficient intake: fruits, vegetables
- Accumulated metabolic waste-acids (from years of eating excessive meats and carbohydrates, and lack of exercise)
- Estimate the ratio of foods eaten. Generally, eat the following *approximate* ratio of foods for your health:

50% <u>Alkaline-ash</u> foods *(fruits, salads, vegetables)*

50% <u>Acid-ash</u> foods *(complex carbo-hydrates like starches, grains, cereals, breads, flour products; and proteins)*

Approximate your food ratios. On any particular day, it does not matter if one meal is mostly alkaline, and another mostly acid—just try to balance it out for the day! If you get it wrong, try again tomorrow. It is a subjective call that you make, and it is what you do over weeks, months, or years that make the difference—not on any one or two days or weeks.

———

Note - If Vegetarian

As a general indication, if you follow a vegetarian diet substitute vegetable sources of protein for the any flesh in the food guide. Note that contrary to most alkaline-ash vegetarian diets you need something different:

*You need an **acid-ash** vegetarian diet high in complex carbohydrates and vegetable proteins.*

Because of your high need for protein, you usually require a daily vegetable powdered protein supplement in juice (about 25-30 grams).

———

Important

- Minimize white sugar and alcohol intake.
- If desired, interchange lunches for dinners.

- Never eat foods you are allergic to, no matter what I recommend; if allergic, or suspect a food allergy, eliminate it and substitute from your type mineral lists.
- Eat the right foods 80-90% of the time and the Food Guide will work for you; unlike some types you do not have to live out of a health food store (although such foods are healthier for you).

▶ *Omit eating the excessive minerals in your type chapter, and be sure to eat one or two servings from the deficient list daily.*

Finally, in addition to your body type needs, other holistic healing matters also need your attention. I strongly suggest that you refer to my web site and earlier books for that information: *DrStenbeck.net*

———

Acid/Alkaline Genetics Chart

The following chart reflects each Muscle Type needs for acid or alkaline-ash foods. These ratios change if you are unhealthy or over age 45-50. Refer back to your body type and review the *Acid/alkaline* instructions.

———

Acid/Alkaline Genetics, Dietary-Ash, and Raw Food Needs

This chart shows the Rocine types, their acid or alkaline food needs, and the percentage of raw foods needed for your health and healing.

- Apply your Type Minerals to the Food Guide

Type Genetics	Acid/Alkaline Needed	% Food-Ash Needed	% Raw Food
Calciferic	Alkaline	70% acid	30
Carbogenic	Alkaline	50-50	50
Desmogenic	Alkaline	70% acid	50
Eldic	Intermediate	50-50	50
Medeic	Intermediate	50-50	50
Myogenic	Intermediate	50-50	50
Nervimotive	Alkaline	70% acid	50
Nitropheric	Acid	70% alkaline	70
Pallinomic	Alkaline	50-50	30

The above percentages vary depending on aging and the health of individual types.

Muscle Types / Food Guide
Breakfast

Use the nutritional information from your Type Chapter everyday in this Guide.

EGGS* (1-2) with lettuce, tomato, or salad, whole grain toast; (add bacon or sausage 1-3 times weekly if desired) — 2-4 times/week; or

FRUIT fresh salad, and protein (yogurt, milk, cheeses, seeds, nuts) —1-3 times/week; or

CEREALS, with fruit, seeds, nuts —2-5 times/week; or

OTHER choices — 0-1 times weekly

<u>*Daily liquids:*</u>
Pure water, citrus, vegetable juices, soups, other —as desired
Coffee, teas —0-2 cups

Muscle Types / Food Guide

Lunch

SALADS, *mixed green, protein (poultry, fish, egg, cheese, seeds or nuts, etc.), whole grain breads [Dressing: olive oil/ vinegar; low-fat, low-cal dressings] — 2-4 times/week; or*

SANDWICH, *whole grains with a protein (cheese, tuna, ham, etc.); and salad and/ or vegetables — 1-4 times/week; or*

POULTRY, FISH, *3-6 oz., with a mixed green salad and/ or vegetables —1-3 times/week; or*

OTHER *choices (with salad or vegetables) —1-2 times/week*

[Other oils are permitted, but less ideal: soybean oil is a common allergen; minimize commercial dressings. Be sure to include two or more selections from your type food lists in your daily food intake. For in-between meal snacks, eat fruit or vegetables with seeds/ nuts.]

Muscle Types / Food Guide
Dinner

POULTRY, FISH *(4-6 oz.), with salad and/or vegetables*
—2-4 times/week; or

PASTA *with protein (chicken, etc.) with salad and/or vegetables*
— 2-4 times/week; or

VEGETARIAN *meal with salad and/or vegetables*
—1-3 times/week; or

LEAN BEEF *(4-6 oz.) with salad and/or vegetables*
— 0-1 times/week

OTHER *choices with salad and/or vegetables*
— 0-1 times/week

Desserts:
Fruits, fresh —as desired
Low-sugar, healthy desserts
— 0-3 times/wk

Food Guide Notes

Steamed Vegetables —

Minerals are lost in the boiling of vegetables; steaming or wok cooking is best.

Food Combinations —

If you have a weak digestive system then eating proteins at the same meal with starches often results in indigestion, gas, or constipation.

Periodic Detox —

You tend to over-indulge in acid-ash foods (proteins and carbohydrates), and often need occasional elimination diets for tissue waste-acid removal. Have a holistic doctor or nutritionist supervise such detox (where you have an alkaline-ash diet along with protein supplementation).

Minimize —

- Fatty foods
- Commercial salad dressings
- Beef, red meats, processed meats
- Coffee, white sugar, corn syrup, alcohol

Vegetarian Proteins —

You require a carnivorous diet. The exception is the *nitropheric* type who functions best with a *vegetarian* diet; the other muscle types are born to be carnivores. It is very difficult for the other muscle types to be pure vegetarians because of their strong intuitive cravings for fish, poultry, meat, or eggs. If you are vegetarian, then because of your high needs for amino acids and acid-ash foods, you should take a protein supplement of 30-40 grams/day (powdered protein in juice).

Healthy Weight —

Several of you gain weight as the ravages of age, lack of exercise and dietary excesses take their toll. By eating according to your body type, you should naturally lose excess weight. Each type also has a few individual factors that only apply to them!

You have a good ability to lose weight by following the Food Guide instructions. The most common problem I find with your weight-control is liver and kidney irritation due to food allergies, which results in extra pounds. The key is to eat non-allergic foods.

If drinking more than 3-4 cups daily of coffee or tea, you may have a hypoglycemic problem (low blood sugar), which contributes to making fat, ill-health, and delayed healing. (Refer to the earlier books for help with this healing.)

———

In some *Fat* types like the lean or medium-sized (when young adults) *isogenic and pargenic*, you may be inclined to call them *Muscle* types: study them carefully to discern the differences.

* * *

Appendix

Brief Extracts from
<u>The 22 Unique Body Types</u>

Appendix A

Types
(Brief extract)

Type comes from 'typus' meaning an image or impression, the study of types being called typology.

▶ *Rocine: "A combination of mental and structural features is consistently found in people of the same type."*

Rocine wrote that all types are a mixture of positive and negative qualities. He based his work on the biochemical individuality of our *mineral* absorption and utilization. Of course, all minerals are absorbed, but he postulated that different types of people *selectively* absorb certain minerals, to a greater or lesser extent, requiring specific mineral foods for their enhanced health and healing.

▶ *The type information cannot predict what or who you will become, or how successful or not, but your type is capable of bringing a creative excellence to whatever you do in life. If your type has negative qualities that you disagree with, remember that they are only tendencies and may or may not manifest in you.*

This book enlarges on Rocine's premise (early 1900's), integrated with the later research of Herbert Sheldon, M.D., Ph.D., at Harvard University (1930's), along with my fifty years of observations and experience with this subject.

Comparing your shared physical (and sometimes psychological) descriptions with the Celebrity Lists further assists the identification of your type. It is not that you will look exactly like, or be a twin to, any particular celebrity. Look closely at a celebrity's features: face, profile, height, weight, head, etc. If you know something about their talents, beliefs, success and failure spheres, health and weight challenges, attitudes and behaviors, etc., then you get clues as to what your type may be.

————

Understanding Types and Sub-Types

Each of us has a clearly discernible dominant type. Visualize the celebrity examples from movies, politics, sports, the arts and public life, and try to identify with their physical features. Look for similar features, remembering that you will not recognize all attributes in yourself. You are not looking for your twin!

The sub-type issue is the main reason people of the same major type can look so different. Remember that a type description does not characterize you exactly, but depicts your individual variant of a type.

▶ *The type questionnaire pinpoints the major features of that type: if the celebrity examples are unhelpful, you may be an unusual variant (in which case ignore the celebrity issue and give yourself 7 points on Question 1).*

―――――

Minerals

Minerals are essential life nutrients that accelerate enzyme and chemical reactions and provide a basis for your body typing. Although found in all tissues, different minerals tend to be concentrated in certain organs, their presence or absence contributing to the healing of such tissues; e.g., zinc accelerates prostate healing; calcium and manganese promote bone, joint and connective tissue healing.

Specific foods nurture each type, some people needing meats for their health others needing a vegetarian diet. A high potassium diet nurtures one person, while another needs high sulfur, calcium, zinc, or another mineral.

Mineral Digestion and Absorption

Compared to vitamins, minerals are *difficult* to digest, absorb, and utilize. In people with strong digestive systems, this aspect may not be important. The following factors should be in place for optimal mineral metabolism:

1. Stomach Hydrochloric Acid Production
2. Parathyroid Hormone Balance
3. Organ Toxic Metal and Chemical Removal
   [See details in <u>The 22 Unique Body Types</u>.]

———

Total Body Healing

Note that from a holistic healing perspective, in addition to minerals and type information, the following healing factors are necessary:

> *Nutrient Balance*
> *Mental Balance*
> *Emotional Balance*
> *Spiritual Balance*
> *Detoxifying Integrity*

The above factors are all important to your total healing especially if you are interested in self-healing (see my earlier books).

———

Appendix B

Researchers
(Brief extract)

The predominant workers in this area of human individuality from around 1880's to the 1960's are Herbert Sheldon, M.D., Ph.D., Roger Williams, Ph.D., and Victor Rocine, D.Sc.

Much information on Sheldon's research exists on-line and in medical psychology libraries; for interested readers there are other lines of research published in the last century. This present book is primarily about Rocine's body types.

Herbert Sheldon M.D., Ph.D.

In contrast to Rocine, Sheldon at Harvard University in the 1930's was trained in the scientific method and did painstaking research and publishing on human individuality. In comparing his findings with Rocine's work, a direct putative correlation is visible.

Roger J. Williams, Ph.D.

Another significant researcher in human individuality is the renowned scientist and biochemist, Roger J. Williams. He demonstrated that different people have varying levels of nutrients, enzymes, and other metabolic chemicals in their bloodstreams.

▶ *Williams's research firmly expands on the premise of individual nutritional needs in human beings. If interested in his research, I highly recommend his book Biochemial Individuality.*

Victor Rocine, D.Sc.

Note that when a negative feature is indicated, say neurotic tendencies, all members of the type are <u>not</u> that way; it is a type tendency reported by Rocine.

Rocine studied type-related diseases finding links between mineral and dietary factors with individual types and their diseases. In each body type, one or more dominant minerals are preferentially absorbed and utilized over other minerals.

He recognized discrete body types from their physical appearance finding genetically based mineral dominance to be the determining feature. He also correlated their physical features with psychological characteristics.

———

Appendix C

Genetics, Types, and Diet
(Brief extract)

This section deals with how nervous system genetics helps determine your eating choices for health: you are either born to be a predominant meat eater, a partial or complete vegetarian, or something between the two. The genetic factor determining this dietary aspect is the *sympathetic and parasympathetic* components of your central nervous system. This represents a basic factor in eating for health.

This chapter helps you understand your dietary inheritance, although instinctively, you may already have arrived there!

- If born **sympathetic** dominant you are *genetically acid*, desiring a predominantly *vegetarian* diet for your health (about 70% fruit, salad, vegetables to 30% proteins and carbohydrates).

- If born **parasympathetic** dominant you are *genetically alkaline*, desiring a predominantly *carnivorous* diet for your health (about 70% proteins, carbohydrates to 30% fruits, salads, vegetables). Few of you ever choose to become vegetarian because of the difficulty in satisfying your protein needs without meats.

- If born ***intermediate*** dominant you may eat food groups with little concern for the acid/alkaline factor. However, after age 40, you need a semi-vegetarian diet for healthy eating.

———

Chart of Relative Nervous System Dominance

In the following Chart, if you relate to many of the symptoms on one side you probably have that nervous system dominance; relating to both sides indicates *Intermediate* dominance.

If Vegetarian (Over-acid) --
Eat 70% fruits, salads, vegetables
And 30% proteins, carbohydrates

If Carnivore (Over-alkaline) --
Eat 70% proteins, carbohydrates
And 30% fruits, salads, vegetables

If Intermediate --
Eat 50:50 of acid and alkaline-ash foods

Make an *approximate* estimate of your daily acid and alkaline food intake (such ratios varying from type to type).

———

Symptoms of Relative Genetic Dominance

Vegetarians (Over-acid)	Carnivores (Over-alkaline)
Sympathetic Dominance	Parasympathetic Dominance
little or no flesh desire	desire flesh
easily constipated	rarely constipated
slow digestion	fast digestion
easily dehydrated	not dehydrated
strong thirst	low thirst
pale face	flushed face
high pulse after food	slow pulse after food
easy gag reflex	slow gag reflex
cool dry skin	moist warm skin
nervous stomach	calm stomach
little eyelid blinking	much blinking
nervous tendency	mostly calm
slower healing	faster healing
low oxygen-uptake	good oxygen-uptake
easily breathless	seldom breathless
insomnia common	sleep easier
few muscle cramps	some night cramps
calcium deposits rare	get calcium deposits

Appendix D

Help Identifying your Body Type with Dr. Stenbeck

If you desire help in identifying your body type, follow these instructions, and answer the questionnaire. For further information and fees, send me an email from page one of the website:

DrStenbeck.net

First name: _____

Country of birth: _____

Upload photos and send to the above website:

- Head and shoulders: front and side views

- Full body: front and side views

- Also 1-2 teenage views

- If possible, casual photos of mother, father, siblings

MY TYPE CLASS MAY BE: _____

   (Thin, Muscle, or Fat)

AGE   - _____

HEIGHT   - _____ feet/inches

MY WEIGHT - _____ pound

- Heaviest age: _____

   - Lightest as adult: _____

   - Estimate age 15:   _____

VISION - Excellent Average   Poor:

HAIR -   Natural color: _____

   - Thin/thick?   _____

   - balding?   _____

SKIN - Quality: _____

   - History of acne, boils, other:

   _____

   _____

TEETH   -   Strong   Weak   Dentures

 - Cavity history: Many   Moderate   Few

MUSCLES -   Strong   Average   Weak

      Sports played _____

JOINTS -   Strong   Average   Weak

HEALTH - Childhood diseases?

   _____

   _____

   - Adult diseases?

   _____

AVERAGE DIET

- Beef _____ (times/week)

- Poultry _____ (times/week)

- Fish _____ (times/week)

- Eggs _____ (times/week)

- Water _____ (glasses/day):

- Vegetarian? Vegan? _____

- Other? _____

- Did your childhood diet differ? _____

The above will help me know who you are! I will send you a follow-up questionnaire for further help in identifying your body type.

Appendix E

On-line Health Consultation with Dr. Stenbeck

For further information, or to comment on this book, or to receive a response on any health issue from a holistic viewpoint, send an email inquiry from page one of my website:

DrStenbeck.net

Following that, I will suggest further healing needs, which we may pursue with an on-line consult.

———

Appendix F

Notes

See my book <u>*The 22 Unique Body Types,*</u> available at the usual online source, for further information and details on all of the 22 Types. The Appendix in that book has further information about:

Mineral Functions and Food Sources

Further Reading

———